Hope is a waking dream.

Aristotle

Healing Perspectives ...

"*Maze of Life* charts a course for us to follow from a world all too often plagued with doubt and fear to one filled with health and HOPE."

- Ronald Fountain, EDM
The Weatherhead School of Management
Case Western Reserve University

"Traveling through the *Maze of Life* is an incredible healing journey. It demonstrates the power of the *human spirit* to remove the obstacle of 'change' so we can begin to heal ourselves."

- Lee S. Berk, DrPH, MPH
Associate Director
Center for Neuroimmunology
School of Medicine
Loma Linda University

Maze
of Life

CONTENTS

Introduction

Three things in life are certain. The first two are obvious: death and taxes. The third, however, is rarely recognized. It is called "change."

Change affects us in many ways. In fact, everything in life is constantly changing: our relationships, jobs, interests, and our health.

In our quest to inspire individuals to maximize their health, two important questions continue to surface. The first is, "How can we help people deal with change?" The second addresses what may very well be the primary issue underlying our healthcare crisis— "How can we help each other embrace change and develop healthier lifestyles?"

We are convinced that each of us has the capacity to develop healthier lifestyles— especially when faced with our mortality. The power of the human spirit is limitless. We can learn to heal ourselves.

The time-tested insights presented in *Maze of Life* serve as a guide for our patients at the Mind-Body Wellness Center who have shared some of their most precious lessons with us.

Their experiences have taught us a great deal. We've observed a number of people who gave up on themselves, and died of potentially curable illnesses. We've also witnessed countless others facing supposedly incurable diseases, given 6 months to live 10 years ago, who are still thriving, and living full and meaningful lives.

They have demonstrated the incredible power of the mind-body-spirit connection— a critical link that should never be underestimated.

Maze of Life, however, is not about avoiding death. It is important to realize that succumbing to an illness is not a failure when we bring back into our lives what is personally healing.

The late Norman Cousins summed it up best with his statement, "Beliefs are biology." What we think and feel becomes our biology, chemistry and immunity. What affects our minds directly impacts our bodies, and visa versa. Stress clearly makes us more susceptible to illness. Developing a sense of purpose, taking charge of our lives and building nurturing relationships strengthen our defenses. Mindfulness, laughter, exercise, proper diet, imagery, music and spirituality have all been shown to promote healing.

There is a growing body of credible medical research that describes the impact of our emotions on heart disease, cancer, diabetes and many other serious medical conditions. Well-respected scientific studies performed at world-renowned institutions clearly demonstrate that we can positively influence the quality of our life and survival when we make healthy lifestyle changes.

Maze of Life is far more than a story about illness. It presents a soul-searching series of questions that only we, as individuals, can answer in order to reestablish meaning and purpose in our lives. It is a journey to be traveled by each of us in our own special way and on our own terms, whenever the need arises— hopefully before we are faced with the challenge of illness.

For most of us, change is an obstacle— perhaps the greatest source of stress in our lives. Yet, for others, it can be embraced as an opportunity to learn, grow and discover the essence of living life fully, and understanding that when the need arises, the maze appears for us.

The inseparable mind-body-spirit alliance is the glue that connects us to the *Maze of Life*. Built on a solid foundation of spirituality through nurturing, hope and trust, this story reminds us of our capacity to turn seemingly unyielding obstacles into new opportunities for discovering inner peace.

Maze of Life is a testimony to the healer that exists in each of us when we trust our spirituality. It builds upon our inner wisdom and encourages us to take action and responsibility for our lives.

In western society, we often believe that survival equates with success. We also tend to focus on what might have been had we lived our lives differently. *Maze of Life*, however, challenges these beliefs.

With utmost respect for your needs and beliefs, this story is intended to inspire you to personally answer the "questions on the walls." It is our hope that you enjoy your journey through the *Maze of Life*.

Maze
of Life

An Important Call

"Joan Livingston is on the phone, Doctor. She sounds upset and says she really needs to speak with you."

"All right, Sarah. Bring in the chart and put her through."

"Doctor, I really need some answers. I'm sorry but I just couldn't wait any longer for my tests. Did you get them?"

"But Mrs. Livingston, you have an appointment on Monday and we should have all your results back by then. Why not settle down and wait until we have a complete picture?"

"But Doctor, you can't imagine what I'm going through. I *know* something is very wrong. Please don't keep it from me. I really need to know now!"

"Okay Mrs. Livingston, give me a few minutes to sort the tests that just came in."

After rummaging through a seemingly endless pile of records, I found some of her results.

Oh God, not again, I thought. Just as I was about to speak, she broke in.

"You can't imagine what it's like not knowing."

Knowing wouldn't be any better, I thought to myself. "Joan, why not come in on Friday? Sarah will fit you in."

"But, Doctor ..."

Deep down inside, she knew what was wrong. She began to cry uncontrollably. How could I tell her that ...

"Okay, I'll come in on Friday," she resigned.

If only she knew how difficult this was for me as well as for her. It wasn't easy being a physician lately. In fact, it never was. She couldn't possibly imagine how hopeless I felt.

"Joan, are you all right?" I asked in a comforting tone. How could she be? There were no words left inside me to comfort her.

There was also no response— only the muffled crying of a woman facing the inevitable, I thought to myself as she continued to weep.

With a sigh, I reached out to her again. "Joan, are you okay?"

My despair was met with a dial tone.

The Last Appointment

It was finally the end of a difficult day. Actually, it was no more difficult than every day had become in the last few weeks.

I suppose life in general had become a challenge— frustrating, in fact. Overwhelming was more accurate. The remaining follow-up calls for the day would do little to chip away at a never-ending stack of things to do that seemed to pile up more each day. How many more patients like Joan Livingston would I have to face?

I sipped what remained of a cup of tea that was at least three hours old. While reaching for the phone, approaching footsteps from the waiting room broke the silence. The door opened, and in walked a gray-haired gentleman who caught me by surprise.

"Good afternoon, doctor," he said as the door shut behind him. "It's nice to finally meet you."

"Who are you?" I asked.

"Why, I'm Jonathan Spes, your 4:00 appointment," he continued in a pleasant and nonchalant manner.

"But, how did you get in?" I persisted.

"Simply through the door," he said jokingly. "Your receptionist was busy so I just let myself in."

"You're not on my schedule," I stated.

"Why you're on mine," he countered lightheartedly. "It seems like this appointment has been scheduled for ages."

"Alright, Mr. Spes. Sit down, and make yourself comfortable. Why are you here?"

"For a routine check-up," he replied. "You come very highly recommended."

Very highly recommended, I repeated to myself sarcastically. If he only knew this wasn't going to be a longstanding relationship, he never would have come through that door in the first place.

Yet, as I focused on his distinctive features and gentle manner, I was immediately drawn to learn more about the stranger who sat before me.

It still irked me, though, that he wasn't on my schedule for the day.

Spes was of average build and casually dressed. His flowing gray hair added to the soothing nature of his warm smile. Despite obvious signs of aging in a forehead that bore furrows of deep thought and contemplation, he projected an energetic sense of youthfulness and spontaneity. His dark blue-gray eyes were deeply set, and his bushy charcoal eyebrows were the perfect match for a short, neatly-cropped beard. He looked like a typical middle-aged college professor.

"Let's start with your medical history," I began. "How old are you, Mr. Spes?"

"I'm not a day less than 77," he responded.

"Are you serious?" I asked with surprise. "You look like you're in your mid fifties."

"A lot of folks tell me that," he said. "Yet, when it comes from a doctor, I appreciate the compliment."

"You really do look wonderful, especially for your age," I emphasized. "To what do you attribute your good health?"

"I wasn't always healthy," he said. "Thirty-two years ago, I didn't expect to survive."

Neither do I, I thought to myself. "What happened?" I asked.

"It began when I was 45," he continued. "I hadn't been feeling well for a number of months, yet I simply ignored the changes I was experiencing. Life, in those days, had little meaning. Recently divorced, and not speaking to my children, I resented everything about my life. Everywhere I turned, I found myself running into walls. After passing out one day in a New York subway, the cops insisted I schedule a visit with a doctor."

"What did the doctor find?" I asked.

"Not a thing, at least initially," he said. "But he was persistent. After what seemed like endless poking and prodding, I waited anxiously for the results of my tests."

"And what did they show?"

"Precisely what I didn't want to hear," he responded. "He told me I had 6 months to live, and that no treatment would make a difference."

"So what did you do?"

"What would anyone do when handed a death sentence?" asked Spes. "At first, I was in denial. As difficult as my life had been, I couldn't bring myself to believe that this was happening to me. Soon anger set in, and distanced me from the world I knew.

"I hated everything and everyone around me. Then, in what was a last fling at foolishness, I began to bargain with myself. If I only did this or that, I would make it through. Frankly, that didn't last long either. Eventually I became depressed and weaker by the day. Finally, I simply settled back, accepted my fate, and was prepared to die."

As I contemplated his words, the old man's account touched me more deeply than he could have imagined. I knew the pain of his experience, and became lost in his story.

"So one day I decided to call it quits," he continued. "I managed to walk down to the old subway station, or the maze as I called it. I suppose I spent a quarter of my life underground in that prison, back and forth from work, day in and day out.

"I realized my life had become a maze. I had no direction, and there was no meaningful goal in sight. I wasted my energy going from point A to point B, and back to point A again. I felt lost, and anticipated each turn as a wrong one. Every path seemed to lead to a blind alley. I felt hopeless, without any reasonable prospect for surviving.

"As I sat down on the old, creaky, rusted bench in the underground station, I thought about those cold, lonely nights I waited there, lost in my own existence. Staring blankly into the endless procession of streaming lights from the passing trains, I saw my life flickering before me like the final scenes of an old movie that gradually faded into darkness. It was an unnerving blur that literally made my head spin. When the last train finally cleared, I felt drawn to the tracks in the train's wake. And then I knew it was time."

"Time for what?" I asked. Sensing his response before another word was spoken, I leaned back in my chair, closed my eyes, and prepared for what I knew was coming.

"Time to hurl myself onto those endless tracks that would seal my fate," he added. "There was simply no other choice in sight. Yet, just as the train passed, and the dust began to settle, what caught my eye was a poster on the wall across the tracks in the distance that struck me harder than you could imagine. It was a maze with the word 'life' inscribed as its corridors."

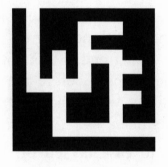

"Life?"

"Yes, Life— L I F E, clear as day," he said. "What could be more ironic?"

"My life had become a miserable, frustrating, and hopeless maze with nothing but a dead end in sight. What a fitting end, I thought. Amidst the graffiti and chaos, there before me was the final writing on a filthy wall. The maze of life, how appropriate a sign?

"Managing to ease myself off the old bench that would never support the likes of me again, I stepped toward the edge, and took one final look at the maze I so despised. I leaned forward, felt faint, and lost my balance."

A Twist of Fate

I felt a hand on my shoulder that jolted every cell in my body. What I expected were the pearly gates; what I saw was a pearly smile.

"Give me your hand, Jonathan," she said in a gentle manner that was curiously soothing. "You seem troubled."

"It's more than trouble I'm facing. It's the end of what's been a miserable life."

"How do you know?" she asked, as her hands firmly supported my trembling shoulders.

"It's the *real* writing on the wall— the final decree, the end of suffering."

"How can you be so sure?" she responded.

"Because I'm dying, or perhaps I'm already dead. Anyway I look at it, there's no hope."

"There's always hope," she countered. "All of God's creatures are either living or dying. It's simply a matter of perspective. Why not consider that ..."

We become
what we set out to be.

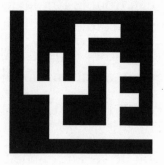

"And I set out to end it all. It wasn't my choice that my life turned out this way. What do you know?" I lashed back.

Unshaken by my verbal attack, she quietly responded, "Sometimes, we're not aware of how or why things happen. Yet that shouldn't stop us from believing we can positively affect our lives. I'm here for you. I'm willing to help you, for I am Hope."

"So where were you when I needed you?" I mumbled under my breath. "You can't know what I've been through. When I was young, I spent years struggling through what had become the maze of my life. I hardly really knew my parents. They were always so busy working, and no one seemed to care. I didn't do well in school, either. They said I had potential, but I simply didn't apply myself. Actually, I never cared."

"I did have friends in high school, though. Those were the only good years. Too bad they didn't last. My friends moved away or went off to college. Again, I was alone.

"I picked up some odd jobs over the next few years, and eventually found a decent job. I reliably showed up every day along with the other guys. At least, it was steady work.

"Three years later, I fell in love, or at least thought I did. The marriage didn't last and she got custody of our children.

"Eventually they eliminated my job— the work I loyally showed up for over the last 20 plus years. They said it was downsizing, and I should have seen it coming. Frankly I didn't. It was a real blow.

"Losing my job was the straw that finally broke the camel's back. I felt worthless and became more bitter with each passing day.

"A month later, one of my co-workers showed up. He said he found a new job that had room for growth. He explained that his manager was a regular guy, and that there was a spot for me if I wanted it."

"What did you do?" Hope asked.

"I turned him down," I said. "There was no way I was about to learn a new job. It was so unfair, and I was so angry.

"I had always been a good employee. Even when there were rumors of the cutback, I showed up early, and stayed late. They just never appreciated my work. I didn't want a new job. I wanted my old job back!"

"So what happened?" she asked.

"I gave up on myself. The rest was all downhill.

"Then one day, while rummaging around the subway, I passed out cold. No surprise, I hadn't eaten a square meal in quite some time. The cops picked me up, and thought I was drunk. The alcohol test was negative, and I awoke in the City Emergency Room. They gave me an injection, and told me to show up at their clinic the following day for additional tests."

"And what did they find?" Hope asked.

"They didn't find a picture of health," I responded sarcastically. "The rest is history, or maybe 'obituary' is a better word. They gave me 6 months to live, no chance for recovery, and a get out of jail free card. At least, I didn't get arrested."

"So what did you do?" asked Hope.

"The only thing I knew how to do," I shouted angrily. "I sulked, complained, ranted and raved, got depressed and nearly starved to death. In fact, the last thing I remember is … I decided to end it all. It was such a blur. My head was spinning. It was so confusing. I was looking down at the tracks."

I paused for a few seconds. "Am I dead?"

"This place is a maze," I said. "I didn't expect heaven to look like this. Or is this hell? Perhaps it's just an extension of the hell I'd been living all my life."

"It's neither heaven nor hell," said Hope. "It will become what you decide it should be. It's your choice."

I thought to myself for a moment. I felt so sick inside and so weak. Everything hurt. But I also felt her hand on my shoulder a few minutes ago. I struck my fist against the wall, and it stung. I must be alive.

"Why did you save me?" I asked.

"I didn't save you, Jonathan. What happens to you depends on you."

"It's not my fault I'm here. Good old fate knocked on the door, and handed me a death sentence!"

"You mean an opportunity," responded Hope.

"An opportunity? Are you kidding? Is this some kind of a joke? Do you consider a death sentence an opportunity?"

"Of course," she said. "It's a chance to put back into your life what has been missing all along. When faced with your mortality, new options for living life fully become apparent. Death is inevitable for all of us. Yet ..."

It's the way you choose
to live your life that counts.
Ultimately, it's a matter of choice.

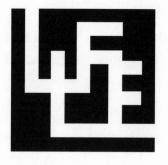

"Are you asking me to choose?"

"I'm asking you to trust your inner voice," Hope said. "Only you know what's right for you."

"What does trust have to do with it? I don't have an inner voice. I spent my entire life wandering aimlessly. What makes you think I can find my way now?"

"Only you can decide what's best for you," Hope said calmly. "I will journey at your side if you so choose. I am here for you."

What did I have to lose? I said to myself. I'm already lost in the maze.

"So how do we begin?" I resigned, in a muffled tone.

"With a first step," she said. "Every journey begins with a first step."

Her words caused something inside me to stir with a sense of energy and warmth I didn't recognize. The feeling was so foreign to me. It was the only spark of anything other than pain I'd felt in months. Maybe she was right, I thought. Perhaps making it through this maze is up to me. It could be that ...

Healing begins within.

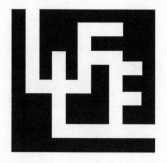

The First Step

"And what is the first step?"

"It is the realization that each of us has to take an active and meaningful role in our own healing process," Hope responded.

But I've already seen the writing on the wall, I thought to myself.

"Jonathan, remember the last thing you saw before you let go?" she asked.

"You mean that poster of a maze with the word 'life' inscribed as its corridors?"

"That's precisely the maze we're about to travel," she said.

"How is it possible?" I asked.

"You begin by traveling with me to a place where healing begins. It is a journey to discover the answers that are buried deep inside you, Jonathan."

"Answers?" I asked in a bewildered tone. "I don't even know the questions."

"Trust me," Hope said. "This maze will provide the questions."

The Journey

As she helped me to my feet, an unsettling feeling stirred within. Wobbly and uncertain, I leaned on her as each step seemed like my last. To my amazement, there was a new path before us.

It was immediately apparent that this maze was strange. The walls radiated with a soft glow, while the floor cushioned every step, unlike the maze I'd been lost in before. The air was fresher as well, and there was a gentle breeze so different from the stench of the maze I attempted to escape.

I also felt different— lighter and somewhat more secure, despite the realization I didn't know where I was going. The further we walked, the easier it became, a feeling so inconsistent with the exhaustion that had consumed me when I prepared to die in the subway station.

"Your first question is before you," Hope said, her words breaking the silence and my train of thought.

I looked ahead, and sure enough there was writing on the wall. The words were not fixed, but seemed to float a few inches from the surface.

How do your beliefs affect your biology?

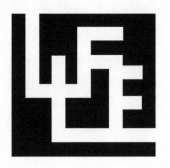

I stopped and repeated the question to myself.

"If I knew the answer, I wouldn't be dying, would I?" I mumbled under my breath in a mocking tone.

"The answer is within you," reassured Hope. "Just stop and think for a moment. What is it you are believing at this very moment?"

"That I'm going to die," I responded in a reflex sort of way.

"Precisely!" declared Hope. "You're telling your body you are not going to make it. Your belief is becoming your biology. It's only natural for every living cell to follow your mind's direction. When you settle for death, your body doesn't argue!"

"You mean ... I can control what goes on in my body?"

"Of course," she said without the slightest hesitation. "It's simple ...."

Beliefs are biology.

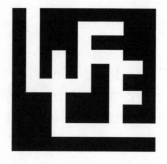

"When you're distressed, your immune system breaks down."

"Wait! Are you saying that when I begin to see things in a positive light, my immune system will bounce back?" I interrupted.

"While a number of factors affect immunity, we each have the capacity to move our immune system in both positive and negative directions. The choice is yours. When the glass is half empty, we're likely to become ill. Yet, when the glass is half full, our bodies tend to assume the biology of health. Why not ask yourself two simple questions?"

"And what might they be?" I asked.

"Is your belief based on fact?"

"But the doctor told me I had only 6 months to live!"

"Jonathan, listen to me," Hope said. "Your doctor may be correct about your diagnosis, but no one can tell you how long you are going to live. Survival depends on a number of things."

"So you're telling me my belief isn't based on fact," I uttered reluctantly. "Let's suppose for a moment you're correct. What's the second question?"

"Is the belief you're holding onto serving you well?" she asked.

"It's no more complicated than that," said Hope, as her warmth and sincerity touched a part of me I had forgotten was there.

I collected my thoughts for a moment before speaking again. "If my belief isn't based on facts, and holding onto it isn't helping me, then I'm sabotaging myself."

"Precisely," she smiled.

"It's finally making sense," I responded in a humble tone. "My belief becomes my attitude, which in turn, becomes my behavior, and ultimately ... the behavior of every living cell in my body. So, if I believe I'm going to die, even though it might not be so, I literally kill myself!"

"In a manner of speaking— yes," Hope said. "Every minute of every day, we're in the process of either living or dying. It's simply our choice."

"But the sadness is so overwhelming," I said.

"Jonathan, life is not an ongoing stream of happiness and positive thoughts. Some challenges are difficult to face and often seem overwhelming. There are high and low points in everyone's life. It's okay to feel sad sometimes. Yet, when such feelings begin to determine the way you live, it's time to rethink your underlying beliefs."

"Then I am going to live!" I shouted, creating an echo that resounded through the walls of the maze. "Is that all there is to it?"

"Frankly, no," she said in a somewhat disappointing tone. "You're missing the point. There's far more to living than just telling yourself you're going to survive. Just as your original belief was not based on fact, your new belief should be built on a foundation of truth. Your doctor explained that you have a serious illness. Let's not deny that fact for now. What could serve you better is a healthy and realistic belief."

I thought about her words for a moment. So— beliefs are biology, I said to myself. I've spent my life with the glass half empty, and look where it's gotten me. Yet, Hope is saying that I can turn my situation around by changing my belief. Something deep down inside tells me she's right.

But there are so many uncertainties, I thought to myself. How can I develop a healthy belief when my future is in question? In order to allow a new belief to take shape, my body must be able to count on it.

Finally it came to me. My new belief must be something I can control.

"Hope," I announced. "It's now becoming clearer. My new belief is: **I choose to live life fully each day, and to do so, I will change.**"

"Well done, Jonathan. You are discovering the wisdom that can help you heal yourself. I knew you had it within you."

I accepted her response as a compliment— the first I had heard in the longest time. Her words lifted me, and soothed my pain. Could I be developing the wisdom to heal myself?

Deep down inside, I hoped she was right. Yet, there was one thing I was certain about. I knew in my heart that traveling with Hope surely made it a lot easier to be positive.

"And where do we go from here?" I asked.

"We continue along our journey," she said.

In my enthusiasm to learn more, my heartbeat and pace quickened. Within seconds, I was way out in front of her when Hope's voice suddenly broke my stride.

"Slow down," she called. "Your quest for discovery must proceed one step at a time. Each step and each moment will reveal something you need for healing."

As her words caught up with me, I stopped in my tracks. I spun around to see her, and what immediately caught my eye was the next question:

What is the most important time of your life?

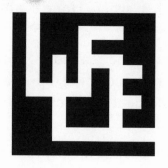

"That's easy," I responded. "It's when I was in high school!"

"Jonathan, why not look at it from another perspective?" Hope suggested. "What you're facing now is nothing less than how you choose to spend the rest of your life, whether it be the next 5 minutes or the next 50 years. What could be more important to you than that?"

"Are you saying my past isn't important— that thinking about the past doesn't help me now?"

"The past no longer exists for any of us, and the future isn't here yet. So, where does that leave us?"

"Nowhere, I suppose. Without my past, I am nothing but a blank slate."

"Jonathan, think about what you just said for a moment. What's wrong with being a blank slate, a fresh canvas, or a new you? What is the only time that matters?"

"Just *now*, I suppose. "I get it …."

Now
is the *only* time
I can help myself.

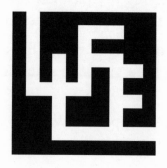

"Exactly," responded Hope. "Many people tend to be very good at living in the past, and some spend a great deal of time preparing for the future. Yet, rarely do we live fully in the present."

"Is that really possible?" I asked. "And how is it going to change my health?"

"Living fully in the moment relieves us of the pressures that stress us and cause us to become ill. We ignore the burdens of the past and the uncertainties of the future. We discover a place within ourselves where worry does not exist, and we rediscover a sense of inner balance."

"And where does that lead us?" I asked.

"To a sense of creating and recognizing what is best for us," Hope said. "That's how you discover what works for you."

"How do I learn to live fully in the moment?"

"Some people practice meditation, or guided imagery, or simply, mindfulness while they walk in the forest. For others, it's an awareness that occurs when they do the things they love like gardening, playing with children, and petting a dog or a cat. It is the full realization that *now* is the best time, the *only* time that really matters!"

I thought about what Hope had been saying, yet I couldn't fully picture what she was really describing. "Hope," I said, "Can you help me get started?"

"Let's sit down for a few moments, and I'll let you experience it for yourself. Allow your eyes to gently close, and focus on your breathing. Know that it's the perfect rhythm for you, and be guided by what comes naturally. Trust yourself, and simply let go. Find a wonderful place deep within, and allow yourself to be there. It might be somewhere you've visited in the past, or just a space you create in your mind. Open your senses fully to take in the richness of the imagery. Picture the surroundings, smell the fragrance in the air, hear every sound, and allow your skin to experience even the slightest sensation. Settle gently into the moment. Be guided by your heart, and listen to your inner voice, as it expresses the truth and the beauty that resides within you. Continue on your own terms, create your own healing moments and savor the joy of your connection with universal wisdom. And when you are ready, open your eyes, knowing that I will be here for you."

After what seemed like a wondrous hour—actually just 15 minutes, I opened my eyes. As my vision cleared, I immediately noticed something different about myself— a sense of inner peace I had never experienced before.

I felt calmer, yet more energized; stronger, yet more fluid in my movements. My vision was clearer and my hearing was more attuned to the sounds in the maze. It was as if each cell in my body was working together for me. Every bit of tension had evaporated, and I felt light as air, yet wonderfully balanced and grounded in a very reassuring way. I realized ...

The imagery I created
had become my biology,
and I felt better.

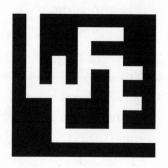

My pain had practically disappeared, and in its place was a refreshing sense of joy. It wasn't about the journey, and it had nothing to do with survival. The most incredible feeling I ever experienced was something so simple: being alive in the moment.

"Hope, for the first time in my life, I don't feel down about myself."

"Jonathan, you're discovering there's no need to judge yourself," she said. "When you learn to appreciate each moment, you free yourself to live life fully."

"I finally understand that who I am and what I'm doing right now is what really counts."

"I agree," she said with a nod and a smile. "Living life fully is not measured in the length of our days. Survival should never be our ultimate goal. It's the quality of each moment that matters the most."

"It is a lifetime of meaningful moments that becomes my future," I said with a great deal of enthusiasm.

"You're on the right track, Jonathan. Just consider this:

You are now creating
healing moments
for your new beliefs
to take hold.

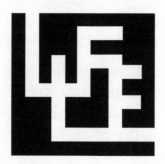

As I continued to walk the maze with a deep sense of calm and awareness, I thought about how much I had learned in such a short time. The maze was evolving into less of a struggle, and more of an opportunity for learning and growing. For the first time in my life, I thought not about the past nor the future, but rather about the joy of the moment.

"Something wonderful just dawned on me," I said to Hope. "Making the most of each moment may be the key to health."

"That's certainly part of it," she responded. "Yet, there's far more to this journey than just living mindfully."

"You mean I shouldn't be living in the moment all the time?" I asked.

"Actually, I'm not saying that at all," Hope said. "Mindfulness is just one part of the healing equation."

As I contemplated her words, another question appeared on the wall ahead.

What is your reason for living?

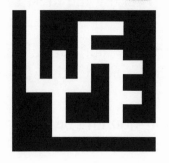

It stopped me in my tracks. I suddenly felt compelled to question all I had learned to this point. Somehow, I felt lost all over again.

While I had gained a sense of hope, a healthy belief and a wonderful tool for discovery, I was taken back by the fact that I didn't even know why I wanted to live. This question struck the core of my being.

"Hope," I asked, "Why is my reason for living important for healing?"

"Understanding your reason for moving onward through the maze is what enables you to discover inner peace," she said. "By answering this question, you discover your purpose in life— why your life is worth living."

"How do I discover my reason for living?" I asked.

"By following the path of your heart," she said. "Only you know what's right for you. No one can tell you how to live your life fully. It can only be done on your own terms when you look within yourself. The tools you are learning to use will help you realize what you need to do. The quest for discovering your reason for living will reveal the key insights you need for healing to occur."

"Hope, how can I go about discovering my true purpose?"

"Jonathan, simply trust your inner voice. Make no decisions until you've contemplated them first. Imagine the outcomes of your choices, see with your understanding, find out what you already know, and you'll discover what's right for you."

"It's something important to think about," I realized. "Something very important I will *always* think about.

"Hope, you've helped me so much. I don't know what I would have done without you and your guidance."

"Just look ahead," she said in a manner that conveyed a sense of knowing what was before us.

As we walked together, I shifted my focus to the wall. What appeared was a question that echoed my deepest thoughts.

How do others affect your health?

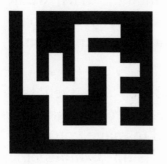

Frankly, before meeting Hope, I never thought much about it. I always considered myself a loner, even when I was married. People never really cared about me, and I'd decided not to care about them either. I told myself over and over that I didn't need anyone in my life.

"Even when I was married, I lived on my own terms," I explained. "Why would I let others affect me? Over the years, some people have made me so angry, even when I wasn't with them."

"That's where forgiveness comes in," responded Hope. "Your negative beliefs created anger that served to make you sick. When you let go of anger, and stop blaming others, you create new opportunities for nurturing. Remember, Jonathan, *they* didn't create your situation. The adversity you experienced with others was precisely what you needed at the time."

"Needed for what?" I interrupted.

"While it's rarely clear to us at the time, the people we choose to be with teach us valuable lessons that help prepare us for the future. Every relationship exists for a purpose," she said.

"Could it be that so many precious moments were wasted ranting and raving? I've spent so much time blaming my parents, my teachers, and even the ones I loved. Sometimes, I even blamed God. It was my fault all along. Hope, I have only myself to blame."

"Jonathan, you have no one to blame— you have only yourself to appreciate," she said. "It's clear that ..."

The process of forgiveness
begins by learning
to forgive yourself.

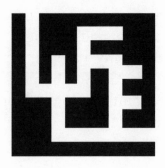

"Forgiving yourself and others are important steps for healing."

"How does forgiveness lead to healing?" I asked.

"When we let go of blame, we remove an obstacle to healing. In doing so, we are set free to grow together, and learn from each other. Through nurturing and support, healing evolves. People who are cared for, and who care about others do far better than individuals who go it alone."

"But it's sometimes so difficult just taking care of myself," I reasoned.

"You're right, Jonathan," she said. "Yet, imagine how much better everyone would be if we supported and nurtured each other. Self-healing also occurs when we give of ourselves, and share our love in the ways we choose."

"Are you saying we depend on others for our health?" I asked.

"In essence, caring about each other builds healthy individuals, families, and communities," Hope responded. "Your gift is to be shared with others."

"What gift?" I questioned.

"It is your capacity to learn, to feel and to create the beauty that's within you when you live mindfully. It is your healing wisdom," said Hope.

"Are you saying that the process of healing myself affects others?"

"Yes," Hope replied. "When we set forth to help ourselves, we positively affect the lives of people who care about us. We also inspire those who share the same very basic needs. Your example illuminates the maze for others."

"Hope, can I help others through the maze, just as you have helped me?"

"Yes," she said. "Yet there's far more to consider, for help alone is not enough."

"What more is there?" I asked.

"It is the way you offer help that matters. It has to be given through choice rather than obligation. Help should be given freely, without strings attached. Some people measure success by what they get out of life. When we see with our hearts, it is obvious that self-worth is based upon a balance between how we give and how we receive. With caring and compassion, healing abounds."

As her words echoed within, I realized this was an important part of my life that needed a great deal of attention. I looked up and beyond Hope, as the next question gradually appeared.

What is the highest form of helping others?

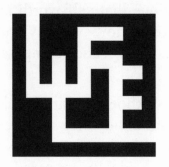

For the first time in the maze, the answer came to me immediately.

"It could only be love."

"Of course," Hope nodded. "Yet there's only so much of you to go around. Saying 'no' is also a healing choice. It's up to you to decide how to share your love. The highest form of helping others is a personal choice reflecting the truth that exists within you."

That realization energized me. I began to walk with a sense of calm and contentment that Hope immediately noticed. We smiled, and continued along the maze together.

Within minutes, the next question began to appear on the wall.

What do you need to do, in order to become whole again?

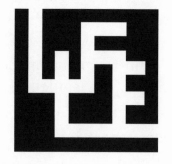

I stopped and thought to myself for quite some time. I was already making healthy progress with a new set of beliefs. I discovered the joy of living in the moment. My purpose in life was clearer than it had ever been before. I realized I had to live every moment fully in order to heal myself. I was already letting go of anger, and was learning to forgive. I felt the wonder of love.

"What more could there be?" I asked.

"Jonathan, you've come such a long way, and I'm so proud of the way you're changing," commented Hope. "Yet, putting into practice what you are learning is the real key to becoming whole again."

"By 'whole,' do you mean living a full and meaningful life?" I asked.

"There's more to it than that," she responded. It's important to realize that ..."

Becoming whole again
is putting back into your life
what has been missing.

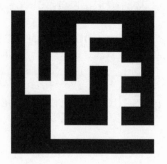

"The problem for many people is that they never recognize what has been lost. Sometimes it's an illness, or even depression that can become a blessing in disguise."

"How can illness or sadness be blessings?" I asked.

"By serving as a wakeup call to a new beginning," Hope said. "I realize it seems harsh."

"Too bad it has to come to that," I murmured.

"It doesn't, Jonathan. Becoming whole is a lifelong endeavor that doesn't require a tragedy."

"I think I understand what you mean. I didn't need this illness to become whole again. Yet, if it wasn't for the diagnosis that nearly ended my life, I wouldn't have found you. I would not have discovered this maze and its particular set of lessons had it not been for my disease. I finally realize the journey to wholeness is an ongoing process, traveled in different ways and experienced one day at a time."

"Jonathan, now is *your* time to become whole again— to rediscover what makes you feel happy and fulfilled."

"It's coming together now. I suppose ..."

I need to take
better care of *me*
so that I can continue
to learn and change.

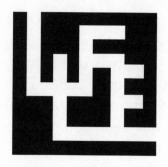

"Belief must become action," she said with a nod of approval. "A healthy way of living enables what's inside of you to heal."

As I thought about her words, wonderful images began to take form on the wall. I saw myself exercising, yet also taking leisurely walks in the forest to feel close to nature. I savored nutritional food, and discovered healthy ways to manage my weight. I imagined enjoying work for the first time in my life, and making time to help others. I also recognized something deeply refreshing within myself. It was a yearning to laugh, to be joyous, and to spend every remaining moment sharing my life with those I love.

Yet, there was something else that caught me by surprise. What excited me the most about living was the opportunity to change.

While no words were spoken, I knew Hope was aware of every thought and insight swelling within me. It was a sense of intuition that exceeded my personal boundaries.

"Where do we ...?" I began.

"... go from here?" she continued. "Yes, I do know what is inside of you, my friend. I've known all along."

Just as I was about to ask Hope to explain, the next question suddenly began to surface on the wall, and it sent a chill throughout my body.

What do you believe in that can restore your health?

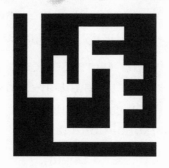

"Hope," I asked. "The questions on the walls are not here by coincidence, are they?"

"Of course not, Jonathan," she smiled. "The writing on the walls has always been within you. There are no coincidences."

"And the questions? They, too, are here for a purpose. I now recognize the words of *my* inner voice— *my* connection with God."

"Yes," Hope responded. "It is your destiny."

"Is my destiny predetermined?" I asked.

"The Creator always places obstacles and opportunities before us whenever the need arises. Actually, they are one and the same. Yet ..."

Our free will determines
how we navigate our mazes.

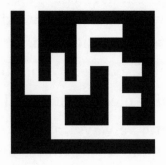

"Are you saying that the corridors of my maze are constantly being shaped by my choices?" I asked.

"Each choice creates new paths and opportunities," responded Hope. "When you begin to see with your heart, you will experience synchronicity."

"Synchronicity, what do you mean?" I asked.

"It is the awareness of what some people refer to as coincidences," she said. "When each of us begins to take better care of ourselves, putting into practice the lessons learned in our mazes, we inspire others to discover inner peace. Their journeys, in turn, affect our lives."

I leaned against the wall, closed my eyes, and relived all the wonderful moments I spent learning and changing with Hope. Finally things fell into place. It was simple now. This journey taught me that ...

When the need arises,
the maze appears,
not as an obstacle,
but rather as an opportunity.

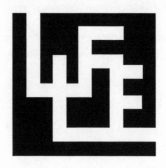

When I was confused, lost and depressed, the maze redeveloped within me for a purpose. It provided opportunities to discover my path to health and well-being.

As I opened my eyes and my vision cleared, I realized the walls of the maze were no longer there. Hope had vanished as well. I stood alone facing an endless horizon— a vast expanse without boundaries. Yet I was paralyzed with a sense of panic and my thoughts began to race.

"Hope! Where are you?" I shouted in desperation. "Please don't leave me now!"

Nothing but the sound of my rapid breathing broke the eerie silence.

I stopped, took a slow deep breath and refocused my attention within. In the stillness of the moment, I began to take control. I opened myself to unlimited possibilities.

Just then, from the depths of my heart, I heard her gentle voice.

"Jonathan, I've always been with you and nothing will ever separate us. We will journey the maze together many times in the future. Whenever your need arises, I will be at your side. For ..."

Hope is the part of you
that comes to life
when you welcome change.

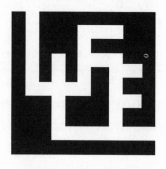

The Doctor's Response

As I looked up at Jonathan, I realized how much his story meant to me.

"Thank you for sharing your story," I said. "I'm pleased that all turned out so well for you. But Jonathan, I mean Mr. Spes, what really happened after the maze disappeared?"

"What replaced the maze was a clear path for living a full and meaningful life," he said. "I simply set off to apply what I learned in the maze. When I began focusing on my answers to the questions on the walls, my life began to change. One step at a time, everything in my life changed— my attitude, my sense of purpose, and my quest for knowledge and growth.

"As I learned to accept my mortality, I realized that …"

Even death would
someday be a change
I could learn to welcome."

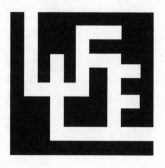

"What did you do?" I asked.

"First and foremost, I decided to live with Hope in my heart. I started taking better care of myself. Soon I began thinking more positively as well. After working and saving enough money, I purchased a bus ticket and moved away from the city. I then worked as a clerk in a wonderful community, and signed up for night classes at a local community college.

"Six months later, I developed the courage to see another doctor. While my original condition hadn't changed, she was astounded by the fact that I was still alive to talk about it. She was open-minded, supportive, and acknowledged that survival was based on a number of factors. The doctor presented some interesting strategies she said were evidence-based. By that, she meant there was a reasonable scientific basis for their use.

"We spent time together figuring out which would be the best choices for me. Within a few days, I began a series of traditional and complementary therapies, and soon I was feeling better than I had in years. I followed her advice, and kept up with scheduled appointments on a regular basis. Five years after receiving a death sentence, I was still alive and thriving."

"And what were you doing at that time?" I asked.

"Believe it or not, I graduated from college with a degree in the humanities, and proceeded to earn a master's degree in journalism. I've traveled the world for the last 25 years, and touched the lives of many people, as they've touched mine. Through many diverse cultural experiences, I've discovered the goodness in all God's creatures, and I continue to share my insights with those in need."

"What do you do for a living?" I asked.

"I simply live the dream. I've discovered the joy of traveling the maze of life wherever and whenever it exists with love in my heart. I spend my life serving as a coach for a number of wonderful people who positively affect the lives of others. Sometimes, I even work as a ghost writer for some very successful authors."

"You seem to have discovered a wonderful sense of meaning and purpose ... and health," I commented.

"I've learned to appreciate life, to experience the joy of laughter, and to bring out the best in people. I've also abandoned fear and embraced change as a way of life," he said.

Seven Questions

As I looked into his eyes, the realization of how deeply his words touched my soul overwhelmed me for a moment. It was hard to believe how positively his story affected me, considering that over the last weeks I had nearly given up on myself.

I looked down at the notes I had taken while he shared his story, and reread the seven questions to myself one more time.

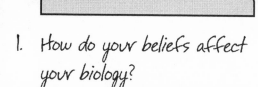

1. How do your beliefs affect your biology?
2. What is the most important time of your life?
3. What is your reason for living?
4. How do others affect your health?
5. What is the highest form of helping others?
6. What do you need to do, in order to become whole again?
7. What do you believe in that can restore your health?

Shifting my focus from the clipboard, I looked at him for a moment, and didn't quite know what to say. Yet I had an uncanny sense he understood what I was feeling.

"Doctor, there's one more thing I'd like to share. It's in my coat pocket in the waiting room."

As he walked out the door, I sat back in my chair and closed my eyes. What more could he share? He had already helped me understand what I needed the most. It was simply the realization that ...

Every moment of life
is precious.

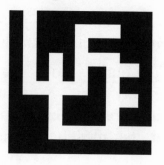

After a few minutes passed, I looked up and listened for sounds in the waiting room. There were none.

I tapped my intercom button, and said, "Sarah, please send Mr. Spes back in."

"Mr. who?" she responded.

"Jonathan Spes, the patient I just saw."

"Doctor, there's no ....

"Are you all right, doctor?" Sarah asked, as she entered the room.

"Sarah, where did Mr. Spes go?"

"Who are you talking about?" she asked. "I've not been away from the front desk all afternoon, and I haven't seen a Mr. Spes!"

"You must have seen him ... gray hair, light-hearted manner, mid-fifties ... I mean seventies. I've been with him for the past hour. He was the last patient of the day," I asserted. "You let him in!"

"But, Doctor, we agreed that you wouldn't see anyone after your 3:00 appointment until you felt better. You needed time to catch up."

"Sarah, he was here. He told me about Hope, and the questions on the walls," I insisted. "He showed me that ..."

We create our own mazes.

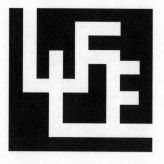

"Look around you, Doctor. I certainly don't see any mazes!"

"He was here!" I declared, as I pushed my chair back into the bookcase.

"Please relax," she insisted. "Everything is going to turn out all right. You probably fell asleep at your desk. It must have been a dream."

"But how could a dream be so real?" I countered. "I knew the man, and sensed his pain."

"Maybe what you felt was your own pain," she suggested. "Your chemotherapy has been difficult for you. But you have a week to rest before your operation. I just know you are going to make it. Everything will turn out okay. Just think positive."

"Positive? Why I've never been more positive. I am positive that I'm going to make it thanks to ..."

I paused and thought to myself for a moment. Perhaps he was a dream, or a figment of my imagination. It didn't really matter. I learned that ...

The opportunity to change is a gift.

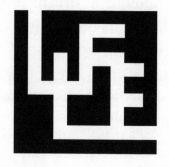

"I suppose I have been working too hard. Thank you, Sarah, for being here for me. You've always been so kind."

"Would you like a ride home, doctor? Shall I call someone for you?"

"Thanks, but I'll be fine. It's been a long day, and it's time for you to go home. I really do appreciate your extra care and concern for me."

As the door closed behind her, I stared at my notes, and rethought what had just occurred, at least in my mind today. Even if it was only a dream, it was a gift, a connection with my inner voice that would never be forgotten.

Real or not, I just discovered a framework for changing my life that resonated with my soul.

In fact, it was more than a message about illness. Mr. Spes showed me how to live my life fully. He inspired me to see beyond illness and he taught me the value of searching within myself for answers that could add quality and meaning to my life.

I now have a healthy perspective for making the most out of my life. Jonathan Spes restored my hope.

Now I realize ...

The mazes existing in all of us
are signs of dis-ease.
When we balance our lives
with happiness and fulfillment,
our path becomes clear.

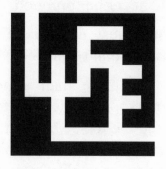

When we become stagnant, depressed, or when we need to change, new mazes appear as opportunities to rediscover the answers that exist within us. What I've learned will be shared with my patients in all phases of their lives— in times of health, during periods of illness and when they are facing the prospect of death.

It's just a matter of synchronicity, I suppose. Jonathan Spes was simply the guide who appeared when I was in need. He provided the inspiration to move onward.

His story showed me how to see with my heart and my understanding. He left me with Hope.

Healing and curing were no longer the same. I discovered healing is a process that enables a person to become whole again. It is far more important than the elusive cure I always sought for my patients to rid them of illness.

Today, this physician trapped in his own maze of pain and suffering discovered a timeless perspective for healing.

I now know ...

When we begin
to take better care of ourselves,
putting into practice the lessons
learned in our mazes,
we inspire others to find their way
to health and well-being.

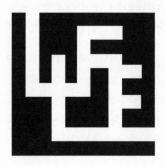

Fear of death no longer overshadowed my life.

As I rose from my chair, something inside felt different. I was lighter, more energized, and in less pain. I recognized a sense of confidence I hadn't known in years.

I will never forget his lessons. At least in my mind, Jonathan had been here with me. Today I became a better person, and a better doctor.

I picked up my jacket, and was about to hit the light switch in the waiting room when something caught my eye. It was a bright yellow envelope on the counter. On it were the words, "To the Doctor from J.S."

A chill radiated throughout my body, causing me to gasp. Alone, amazed and tingling with excitement, I took a deep breath, leaned back against the counter, and held it for a moment in my hands. Then I opened it.

Inside, on a shiny white card was a maze with the word "life" inscribed as its corridors. It read ...

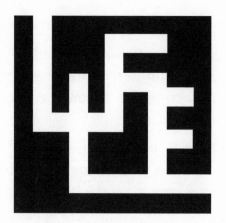

Start Now!
**Discover your path to
health, happiness
and inner peace.**

It was time to visit Mrs. Livingston.

Thank you, Jonathan.

Epilogue

Maze of Life is a story that can help you navigate your own maze whenever the need arises. It should not be considered a road map for living your life, but rather a compass to provide direction for discovering the questions and answers that exist within you.

While we share so many common experiences in life, each of our mazes is unique. Your writing on the wall exists for you, alone. It is not carved in stone— what you need to learn constantly changes as you proceed through your maze.

When challenges surface, the *Maze of Life* appears as a chance to rediscover what has been lost. It provides an opportunity to create changes within yourself and new direction to move onward in your own special way.

People often ask how to get back on track. Some begin by reflecting upon portions of this story that are particularly meaningful for them. You might elect to just review the 7 questions on the walls, or create your own. Many readers have used this short story as a focus for dinner table interaction with their family. Support groups have read this story aloud, thereafter discussing its meaning and relevance from many perspectives. Perhaps, you'll decide to share it with a friend in need.

It's not surprising that life has high and low points— perceived successes and failures. It's only natural to welcome the good times. Yet, hidden within adversity is the opportunity to learn and grow—to become whole again, one step at a time.

It is our wish that you not spend your time looking back at what might have been, but rather looking forward to your maze as a valuable gift for realizing what you want in life.

Allow yourself to anticipate your journey as an adventure and savor each turn in your maze through the wide eyes of the inquisitive child within you. Beyond each corner, new questions, answers and opportunities await you.

Know that at any stage of your life what really matters is within your grasp. You can transform your greatest challenges into a clear path for personal fulfillment.

Additional copies of

Maze
of Life

can be purchased from:

TOUCH STAR
PRODUCTIONS

522 Jackson Park Drive
Meadville, PA 16335
Telephone: 800-759-1294
Fax: 814-337-0699
Internet: www.touchstarpro.com

QUANTITY DISCOUNTS AVAILABLE

About the Authors

Barry Bittman, MD is a neurologist, author, international speaker, award-winning producer/director and inventor. He is CEO and Medical Director of the Mind-Body Wellness Center, a comprehensive, interdisciplinary outpatient medical facility in western Pennsylvania. His medical perspectives have been presented in his book, *Reprogramming Pain,* written to help individuals transform pain and suffering into health and success.

Dr. Bittman has been awarded three patents for his invention, *Mindscope,*® introduced in 1992 as the world's first clinical tool linking the nervous system to a multimedia environment.

His research and "whole person" approach have been featured in numerous publications throughout the world including *USA Today, Business Week,* the *New York Times,* the *San Francisco Chronicle, Men's Fitness, Alternative Therapies* and *Self* Magazine.

Dr. Bittman began TouchStar Productions, a company dedicated to helping individuals harness their inner healing resources as a complementary approach to traditional medical care. His film, *Affirmations For Getting Well Again* won first place awards in the American Medical Association's *1997 International Health and Medical Film Festival* in the categories of Cinematography and Wellness.

Excerpts from TouchStar's features have appeared on nationally syndicated television shows including *Home and Family, CBS This Morning and ABC Nightly News.*

Dr. Bittman is the host of *Mind Body Matters,* the nation's first weekly syndicated National Public Radio show focused on integrative medicine.

He and his wife, Karen, have three children, Benjamin, Marcus and Lauren, and two dogs, Millie and Nala.

Anthony DeFail, MPH is a management expert, author and innovator in the healthcare field. He is currently President and CEO of MMC Health Systems, Inc., a multi-corporation encompassing all facets of health care. With an intense focus on shaping the health care of the future, he is the co-creator of the Mind-Body Wellness Center, founded in 1997. He is also President, CEO and founder of Crawford Health Plan.

Crawford Health Plan has united employers, the hospital and the community through a successful working relationship to manage health care expenses. DeFail's innovative approach resulting in an effective community cooperative has been featured in numerous publications including *Health System Leader*, *Hospitals & Health Networks*, and *Common Goals*.

DeFail, an electrical and biomedical engineer, has 27 years of experience in hospital and community health care, health insurance, hospice and home care. He successfully spearheaded a consolidation of two hospitals into one medical facility. As the CEO of a healthcare system, he has been instrumental in placing his organizations on the cutting edge of medicine and technology by establishing a physician teaching facility with advanced state-of-the-art services— part of a unique combination of resources that is vital to quality health care.

DeFail is a Fellow of the American College of Healthcare Executives and a member of the American Hospital Association, the Hospital Association of Pennsylvania, Alliance Health Network, and the Hospital Council of Western Pennsylvania.

He and his wife, Jane, have two children, Tony Jr. and Alicia.

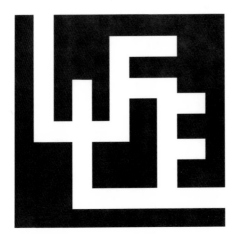

Start Now!

Discover your path to health, happiness and inner peace.

Maze
of Life

Barry Bittman, M.D. • Anthony DeFail, M.P.H.

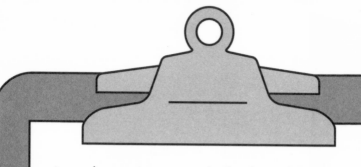

1. How do your beliefs affect your biology?

2. What is the most important time of your life?

3. What is your reason for living?

4. How do others affect your health?

5. What is the highest form of helping others?

6. What do you need to do, in order to become whole again?

7. What do you believe in that can restore your health?